Stress Eating:

How to STOP Using Food to Cope!

Carol L Rickard, LCSW

Well YOUniversity® Publications

Copyright © 2016 Carol L. Rickard

All rights reserved.

ISBN 10: 0-9908476-7-5
ISBN-13: 978-0-9908476-7-0

Stress Eating: How to STOP Using Food to Cope!

by Carol L Rickard, LCSW

All rights reserved. No part of this book may be reproduced for resale, redistribution, or any other purposes (including but not limited to eBooks, pamphlets, articles, video or audiotapes, & handouts or slides for lectures or workshops). Permission to reproduce these materials for those and any other purposes must be obtained in writing from the author.

The author & publisher of this book do not dispense medical advice nor prescribe the use of this material as a form of treatment. The author & publisher are not engaged in rendering psychological, medical, or other professional services.

Disclaimer: The purpose of this material is educational only. Please see you doctor before starting any exercise program or concerning any medical advice you may need.

Well YOUniversity® Publications,
a DBA of WellYOUniversity, LLC
888 LIFETOOLS

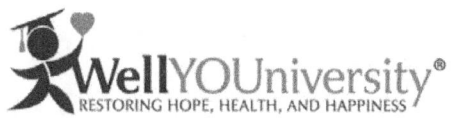

What will you get out of this book?

- Simple tools for making healthy changes in your life.

- Being better able to manage 'waist', *rather than* your 'waist' manage you!

- Improved quality of life!

Stress Eating:
How to STOP Using Food to Cope!

About This Author	1
What It Is & What It Is Not	3
Chapter 1 The "D" Word	4
Chapter 2 Got Tools?	6
Chapter 3 Keys to Changing Your Tools	16
Chapter 4 Get Moving	23
Chapter 5 Why Wellness?	30
Chapter 6 Carol's Laws of Lasting Weight Loss	34
Chapter 7 Is It Really Hunger?	44
Chapter 8 Creating The Release Valves	48
Chapter 9 Stress Management Made Simple	59
Chapter 10 The Power Tools	78
Chapter 11 Wrapping Things Up	99
Chapter 12 A BONUS!	106

About This Author

As you will come to discover, my life has been a journey which has taken me over some **VERY BUMPY** roads.

Along the way,
I have been blessed with opportunities to learn
healthy ways of managing those bumps

&

growing as a result of using them.

Over the past **25** years,
I have taken what I've learned

&

I've been teaching people
how to apply it in their own lives.

Many people have been able to transform their lives.

**My goal is to be able
to help you transform your life!**

This 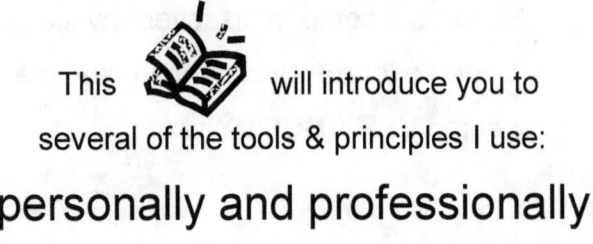 will introduce you to
several of the tools & principles I use:

personally and professionally.

I know they work when put in to action!

If for any reason you are not satisfied

or

feel I have failed to give you tools to transform your life,

I will gladly refund your money.

PLEASE!

If you find yourself benefiting from this material,
Email us at: Success@WellYOUniversity.com
Share your story with me and the rest of the world.

Become a **voice of inspiration** to all the women

still out there struggling to be successful.

What It Is!

This book is like nothing else you may have seen! Along with **simple** easy to understand chapters, I tend to use a lot of pictures, analogies, & word art to make the information stick in the brain!

It is designed to give you tools & knowledge needed to go forward and be successful!

What It Is NOT!

A Quick Fix

You will find **no** "magic pills, exercises, or diets ….

If you are looking for that,

I'm sorry but you won't find it here!

Let me save you some time and suggest you

stop reading right now!

The "D" Word

How many **DIETS** have you been on in your lifetime?

5 10 15 Okay, I'll stop there!
I don't want to give your age away!

Ever tried one of these *'sworn to work'* diets?

The Low Fat Diet, The Carb Diet

The Hollywood Diet, The Grapefruit Diet

The Cabbage Soup Diet, The Beverly Hills Diet

I actually made my own diet when I was in college – the Dr. Pepper & popcorn diet!

How did these diets work for you?!

I guess if they had, you wouldn't be reading this book!

The truth is DIETS DON"T WORK!

There are MILLIONS of women, like us,
who have tried many a diet only to lose **& gain again**!

By the time you get done with the rest of this book – the steps to *successfully managing* your waistline will all make perfect sense to you!

This is my promise to you!

Got Tools?

Do you have a tool box 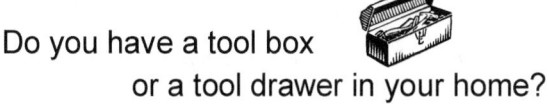 or a tool drawer in your home?

I'll bet money you have either **one or the other!**

Just as we have tools around to take care
of the 'physical' problems in our life,
we also need to have tools around to take care
of the 'emotional' problems in our life..

Now, I have another question for you!

Have you ever taken a knife and
tried to use it as a screwdriver?

Be honest!

(Usually when I ask this question in my workshops,
EVERYONE in the room raises their hands!)

How did it work?

Not *too* well, right?

At some point, we have to come back with
a real screwdriver and fix it again!

Now, just in case you are one of those people who thinks the 'knife' worked just fine –

This question is for you!

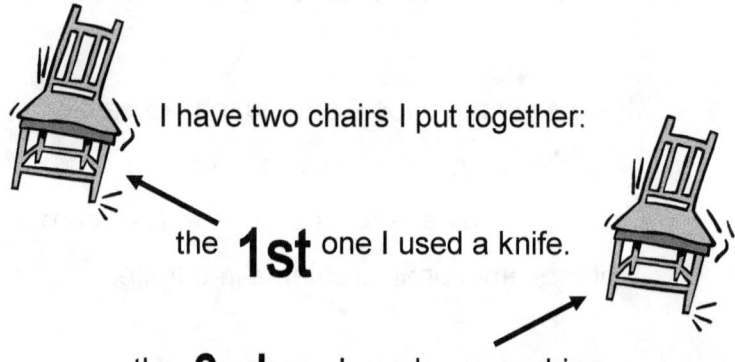

I have two chairs I put together:

the **1st** one I used a knife.

the **2nd** one I used a screwdriver.

Which chair do you want to sit in?!

I *thought so*….. the <u>screwdriver</u> chair!

Let's face it –

having the **'right tool'** for a job

can make all the difference

between **success** & failure.

I don't know about you….

I want to only have to do the job ONCE !

Survival Tools vs. LifeTools

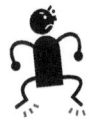 I believe the same kind of situation can happen when we are faced with 'emotional' problems.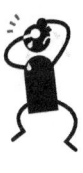

We just grab at something quickly to help us deal with a situation,

I call these **Survival Tools**.

These are all the things we may have used to help us get through the tough times in life.

To help us **SURVIVE** ….

And in many instances,

they do help us – temporarily.

The problem is that many of these
SURVIVAL TOOLS
go on to *become* the problem.

Let me share a couple of examples:

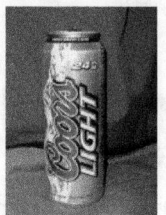

Coors Light is a registered trademark of Coors Brewing Co.

What you are looking at is a picture of one of my old **SURVIVAL TOOLS.**

It was December of 1976 when I overheard a conversation *I wasn't suppose to*. I learned my father was dying from cancer. I was 14 at the time, just in my freshman year at Yosemite High School.

Now, I didn't tell anyone what I had heard…

Instead, I started stealing liquor from my parents. We had just sold a bar & restaurant so there was **PLENTY** of alcohol for me to get my hands on.

Also, my parents were busy dealing with my father so no one noticed if anything was missing.

The truth be told, if my family had known how much I'd been drinking – I know I would have been put in rehab.

Luckily for me, drinking

did not stay my survival tool.

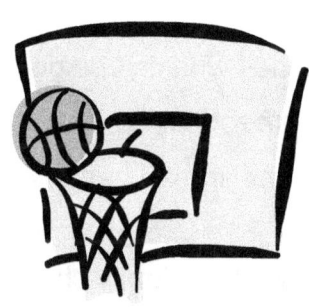

Became my **LIFETOOL!**

You could find me on a court somewhere

shooting for hours on end

&

the drinking came to a stop.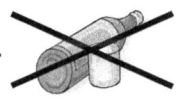

Unfortunately, in May of 1977,

I had a new **SURVIVAL TOOL** emerge –

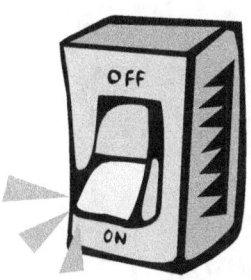

It was 6:00 o'clock in the morning on May 2, 1977.
I had just woken up & was on my way down the hallway to get ready for school when my Mom stopped me.

As she told me I wouldn't be going to school today because *my father had just passed away*, I remember wrapping my arms around her and saying "It'll be okay."

My world instantly changed……..

In that moment, which I can recall as if it were yesterday, I also remember making
<u>a very conscious decision -</u>

I would just go on with my life as if my father had never been there to begin with…..

I flipped my emotions switch OFF.

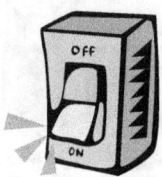

It stayed my **SURVIVAL TOOL** for a very long time

It wasn't until my early **30**'s that I realized what had once helped me **SURVIVE** was now interfering with my life and preventing me from **LIVING**.

It started to interfere with a *very important relationship*.

I had a choice: keep on not dealing with my emotions in a very healthy way or change and learn a new way

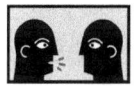 I didn't want to lose the relationship, so I started seeing a therapist for counseling.

I think of counseling as sort of a way to
learn more about yourself.

We don't know what we don't know!

Sometimes we need help from an objective party, outside our family and friends, to help guide us in the discovery to learn more about ourselves.

(I didn't realize the connection between my relationship problems & the emotion switch until I was in therapy!)

What I came to learn is:

Emotions are just like coins –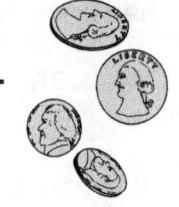

There are
2 sides to them & they can't be
separated!

In order to FEEL joy, love, happiness….
we must also feel sadness, anger, & pain

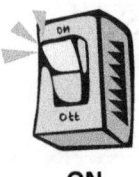

With my emotion switch back on
life has become much richer!!

NOTE: If you can find yourself relating to my story,
and realize you "disconnect" from your feelings,
it may be important for you seek out professional help
to assist you in sorting through the issues & emotions.

There is one more example of **SURVIVALTOOLS**

I want to talk about –

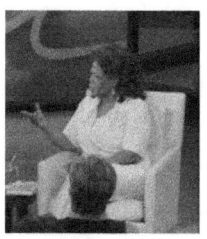

We all know who this is!

It is no secret that Oprah struggled with her weight for many years...

I remember seeing her, in 1988, come out on her show wearing those really skinny jeans, pulling a wagon behind her which represented all the weight she lost.

The success lasted one day!

It took her many more years to figure out **the secret:** she used food as a way of coping with emotions!

I hope by now you begin to have a clearer picture of what **SURVIVAL TOOLS** are & why we need to swap them out for **LIFETOOLS!**

Could FOOD be your SURVIVALTOOL?

Keys to Changing Your Tools!

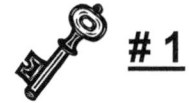 **#1**

YOU are the one who must decide….

If what you're doing in life is working or not?

No one can answer this for you!

The fact remains that no matter what someone else tells us or how hard they try to get us to **change**….

We must make the decision ourselves!

Otherwise,
>*change will be very short-lived*
>***if*** *it happens at all!*

Steven Covey says it best:

"The gate of CHANGE can only be opened from the inside"

 **# 2**

It is important not to *invalidate* the old tools….

I think it is very important **not** to beat yourself up over past behaviors. It doesn't matter if your old tools have been food, alcohol, drugs, sex, work, or anything else

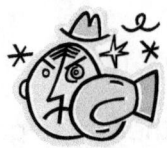

I think it is also very important to validate
the fact these old **SURVIVAL TOOLS**
helped us do just that: **SURVIVE**

I am where I am today because those early **SURVIVAL TOOLS** were a part of my life. Instead of looking at them with guilt & shame, I see them for what they were: some things I '*grabbed at*' to help me get through the **VERY difficult times in my life**

Simply put – they are tools that I no longer choose because I have healthier ones I can use!

 **# 3**

YOU are the only one….

One of my mentor's, the late Jim Rohn has a great line:

"You can't pay somebody else to do your push-ups for you!"

I hate to break the news to you –

<u>We</u> are the only ones that can make these changes!

In order to be successful,

We must take **100%** responsibility!

&

We must **DO**

what we **DON"T FEEL LIKE DOING!**

 **# 4**

Watch out for the COMFORT ZONES!!

One of the greatest **challenges of change**

is that we are

comfortable with what we know.

We must be on the look out & notice when
we are going back to our old 'comfort zones".

Trust me, **this WILL happen**!

The key is to be on the look out for it,
recognize it is happening, and
then take action to get ourselves back on track!

I love the exercise we do in my workshops that helps people to experience this for themselves. I learned it in a training from Jack Canfield, one of the authors of the "Chicken Soup for The Soul" series.
Here's how it goes!

Put your hands together in front of you, interlocking your fingers. (like the picture!) Use left elbow to hold the book open!!

Now, leave everything the way it is but reverse the thumbs so they are the opposite of what they were!

Go ahead and do it now!

How does it feel?

At first, it will feel kind of **uncomfortable!**

You may be *tempted* to go right back to the other way, which feels more comfortable.

Go ahead & resist the urge & hold them in this position! You will notice it starts to feel a little less weird! Hold it even longer and it will actually

start to feel more comfortable.

This is a great way to reinforce what happens to us when we try to make changes in our lives.

It FEELS UNCOMFORTABLE!

We have to keep practicing the new behavior so we start to establish a **new comfort zone!**

Besides the natural tendency to want to stay in our comfort zones, there's one other <u>HUGE</u> stumbling block to making change:

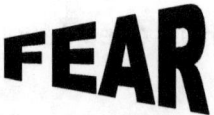

It is said we are born with **TWO** fears:

1) the fear of falling

2) the fear of loud noises

and all the others we learn!

What fears have you learned that you'd like to get rid if?

The next chapter will give you some tools for the job!

Get Moving!

Breaking Through Fear

There are several tools I teach to help my patients bust through fear & make healthy changes in their lives.
I would like to share them with you!
(These are the very same tools I live by!)

"Words can be powerful, put in to action, they become life changing!"

Carol L Rickard

Tool # 1

If you always do
what you've always done,

You'll always get
what you've always gotten,

Because if nothing changes....

NOTHING CHANGES!

Author Unknown

(I think this kind of speaks for itself!)

Tool # 2

One of the best books I ever read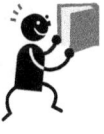
&

the one that helped me really learn to manage my fears:

"Who Moved My Cheese"
by Dr. Spencer Johnson.

If you haven't read this, I strongly recommend it!

It is a short story, about 90 pages long, about these little characters who live in a maze and are forced to deal with change.

It can be a LIFE CHANGER.....

You'll have to look for the book in the *business sections*.

However,

it truly is more of a **Life Lesson's** story!

Tool # 3

It was during the first time I played an audio version of **"Who Moved my Cheese"** for my patients when I came up with this next tool.

I was sitting there, thinking about how to help people **see** change in a different way so they would welcome & embrace it rather than be afraid of it. I came up with:

Creating

Healthy

And

New

Growth

Experiences

© 2016 & licensed by Well YOUniversity, LLC
Taken from "Words At Work"

(The first of many other "Words at Work!")

Tool # 4

While we don't get to control the events in our lives,
We *do get to control* our response to them!
We either **make our choice**
or **let fear** make it for us!

FEAR is NOT an **acceptable excuse!**

We are 100% responsible for our **choice:**

Controlling
How
Our
Intentions
Create
Experiences

© 2016 & licensed by Well YOUniversity, LLC
Taken from "Words At Work"

Tool # 5

Feel the fear and do it anyway!

This is the title of another great book, **"Feel the Fear and Do It Anyway"** - Dr. Susan Jeffries It also is a great tool when you put it in to practice!

There are **2** more strategies I'd like to share:

1) Recognize that fear is really our brain *playing a trick* on us! It may help you to look at fear in the following way: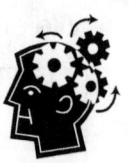

> **F**ind
>
> **E**motion
>
> **A**lters
>
> **R**eality
>
> © 2016 & licensed by Well YOUniversity, LLC
> Taken from "Words At Work"

2) This next strategy is another one I learned from a Jack Canfield training:

You can do this either standing or sitting. Pinch your thumb and 1st or 2nd finger together on both hands.

Hold them out in front and to the sides of you.

Now repeat this mantra in a low 'hum':

"Oh what the heck, go for it anyways"

(If you don't want to make a scene, you can always say it in your head!)

I love this strategy!!!!! One of my favorites!

It's a great way to break through the old fear recording that plays in our head!

I think it works so great because it combines **the mind & the body**...

Why Wellness?

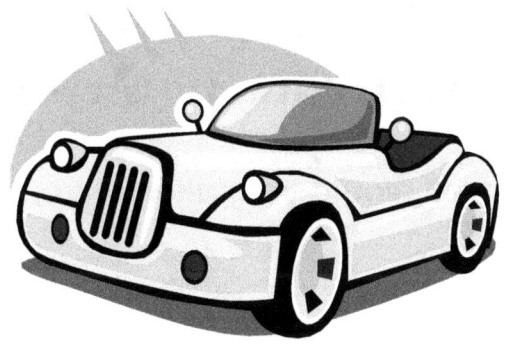

HOW MANY CARS HAVE YOU OWNED?

or

HOW MANY HAVE BEEN IN YOUR HOUSEHOLD?

(This includes new & used ones!)

1

3

5

Maybe More!

(Depending on your age of course!)

Imagine….

You had 1 car that had to last you a lifetime.

How well would you take care of that car?!

If you are like most people,

you would probably take **very good** care of it,

including regular *preventive* maintenance!

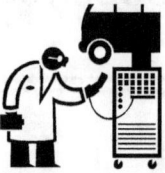

Well, I love to be the one to break the news to you…

We **ONLY** get one vehicle to *live our life with!*

ONE BODY that has to
LAST A LIFETIME!

What is Wellness?

For many years, I used to define wellness as
"optimal health".
I liked the definition because <u>not</u> <u>everyone's</u> the same.

The person who has asthma will be different from the person who does not, yet they can still strive for wellness.

A couple years ago, as I was preparing to deliver a keynote speech in North Carolina, I came across an even better definition. I use this one now, exclusively.

The National Wellness Institute's:
"Wellness is an active process of becoming aware of and making choices towards a more successful existence."

After all, **wellness is the key** to having this **one body be able to last us a lifetime!**

Carol's Laws for Lasting Weight Loss

A Special Note:

Before we get started,
I would just like to say this is the *only* time
you will see me use the word 'weight'!

I don't believe in weight as an accurate measurement.

 I don't own a scale; I never have, & never will,
I also believe you shouldn't either! Here's why:

You see, muscle weighs twice as much as fat...
so even though the scale says
a woman weighs 150 lbs.
she may wear a size "6"!
Or
the scale says she <u>didn't lose any weight</u> YET

she loses 2 sizes in her clothes!

Current health research is now backing this up!
It is our *waist & hip* SIZE that are being identified as
one of the **greatest predictors of our risk for**
heart disease, cancer, and diabetes.

This same research has shown that

if

we *lose* **2** *inches* off the belly,

we significantly **reduce our risk** for the same diseases!

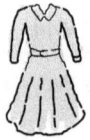 Before you go any further, pick an outfit you would like to have **fit better!**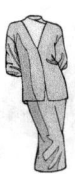

If you still have your eye on the scale,
be sure to **also** pay attention to
how your clothes fit you!

Remember:

it's about us managing our waistline
instead of
our waistline managing us!

Now on to

'Carol's Law's for Lasting Success!!'

Law # 1:

Don't put more GAS in the tank than it can hold!

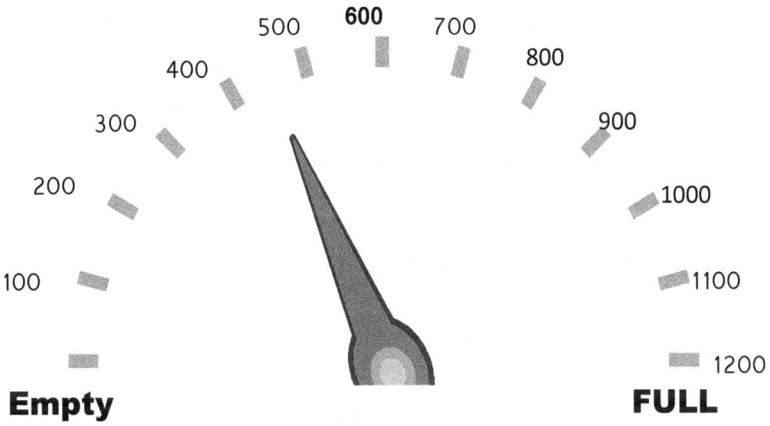

This law makes sense, doesn't it?!

After all, when was the last time you over filled the gas tank in your car? I'll bet NEVER!!!!

When was the last time you over filled the gas tank in your body? Yesterday?!

Does it make sense that just like our cars, our bodies can only hold so much fuel!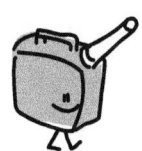

Unlike the car, **our bodies will just keep making SPARE TANKS** to store the extra fuel we're putting in!

Law # 2:

You've got to RUN the engine to use up the GAS!

Think about it!   It really is quiet simple!

Anything requiring movement & muscle involvement is our equivalent of **'running the engine'.**

Certainly, the more often the engine runs,

the more gas that gets used up!

I am not talking about having to go to the health club or gym to accomplish this either.

By increasing your activity levels through out the day, we are ensuring more gas gets used.

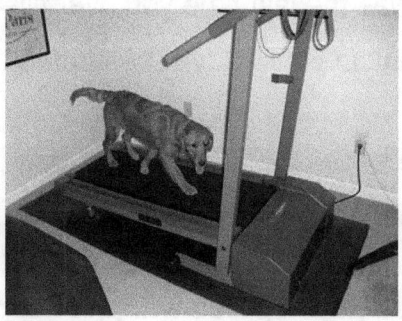

These same laws hold true for dog's too!

Law # 3:

Be careful of which type of GAS you use!

Just as it is important we pay attention to the type of gas we put in our cars; we must also pay attention to the type of fuel we are putting in our body.

It is true that over the years we have been told *all different* types of **recommendations** for healthy eating.

Now they say many weren't so good for us!

Here are a couple of basic "Fuel Rules" to follow:

1) Watch out for "SUGARS"

They can really mess up an engine!

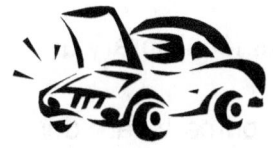

2) Be careful which "OILS" you use!

The wrong ones can very easily clog up the lines.

3) Make sure all "Fuel Additives" used are the right ones for your make and model!!

I didn't go in to detail here because
I *am not a nutritionist*!

I strongly encourage you to do
more studying in this area:

<u>Ways to learn more:</u>

- ✓ Check your local hospital for:
    - o community health education classes
    - o working with a registered dietician

- ✓ Check you local community college for
    - o a non-credit class on nutrition
    - o an upcoming community workshop

- ✓ Check out your local library or big bookstore

- ✓ Talk with your primary care doctor or provider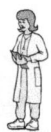

Law # 4:

Use up what we've stored in the SPARE TANKS!

There are two ways we can do this:

A) Be sure we **fill our DAILY tank** *a little less than full*. This way, when we get to the end of the day, we have to use some fuel reserves from the SPARE TANKS!

B) When we fill our DAILY tank to full & **increase the amount of fuel we use by becoming more active** – we will also pull from the SPARE TANKS!

PSS.   If we combine #1 and #2 – we really setting things up quite nicely!

<u>**IMPORTANT NOTICE –**</u>

If we try to pull **too much** or **too fast** from the SPARE TANKS.......

a built-in safety system locks them closed
&
starts to **hold on to more** of the DAILY fuel.

That's why people who eat really low amounts of calories initially lose but then hold on to & **regain** twice as much back.

PS. One of the most frustrating things with this law: we don't get to choose which spare tank it comes from 1st!

And the place we want it to come from **1st** is usually **the last!**

Just means we have to:

<u>'Keep on **Using**</u>

<u>to</u>

<u>Keep on **Losing**!!'</u>

WARNING:

if we're not careful with our fueling practices –

we can end up refilling those SPARE TANKS!

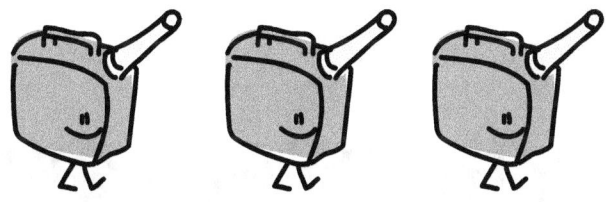

****

The truth to these laws is my life -

I have a friend who always likes to
point out to people I am still the same size as
when she first met me 20 years ago!

I tell her it's because I follow the **Laws of Carol!!**

Now you can too!

I teach and **LIVE** the principles I share with you today!

This is how I know they work!

Is It Really HUNGER?

A Beginning

I believe this area gets paid the *least amount* of attention in our **battles of the waistlines** & the **war on obesity**.

You'll notice in the media & in politics a tendency to focus on nutrition & healthier eating habits along with increasing physical activity.

What we don't see is any real focus on **WHY** people overeat.

I am making it my mission to start a dialogue
&
begin to shift people's focus in this direction.

I want to **thank you** for giving me the opportunity to start a dialogue with you!

Let's keep it really simple & take a look at the following:

There are two types of hunger.

We must start to pay attention & become aware of which one it is that has us eating!

Hunger

Emotional | Physical

Emotional	Physical
Comes on suddenly	Is gradual
Felt above the neck (craving for ice cream)	Felt below the neck (growling stomach)
Must be Certain Food (like pizza or chocolate)	Any food will do (just needs fuel!)
Wants to be satisfied instantly	Can wait
Guilt	No guilt

Source: Researchers from University of Texas Counseling & Mental Health Center

Carol's 2 Steps to Success

1) *Identify the Source*

    Is it physical hunger

        or

            Is it emotional hunger?

2) *Take Action!*

    If it's physical hunger –

        FEED it with healthy choices

    If it's emotional hunger –

        FEEL IT

            &

                RELEASE IT!

Creating the Release Valves

All Shook Up

Has this ever happened to you?
You go into a store & buy either a liter of
diet coke or some raspberry seltzer.

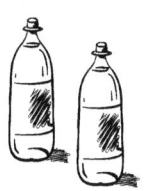

Along the way, you are very careful not to shake it up!

Then one evening that next week,

you go to pour yourself a glass,

your mind busy paying attention to dinner on the stove

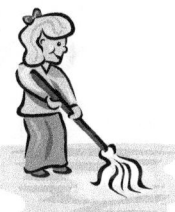

and …….

SPLASH…….

stuff comes flying out of the bottle you just opened -
all over you & the floor creating a mess!

Sometimes in life,

it doesn't matter how careful we are.

Things will still get shaken up!

I believe the same thing happens

when it comes to our emotions!

Sometimes **WE** get *shaken up!*

And if we aren't careful,

we end up with a **BIG EMOTIONAL MESS!**

If we are to have any success at moving away from

using food as a way of coping with our emotions,

then

we have got to learn a little more about

managing them in a healthy way!

I want to introduce you to my system I call

"The Feeling's Pendulum".

Take a look at the next page
& see where you would put yourself!

The Feelings Pendulum

What Do You Do With Your Feelings?

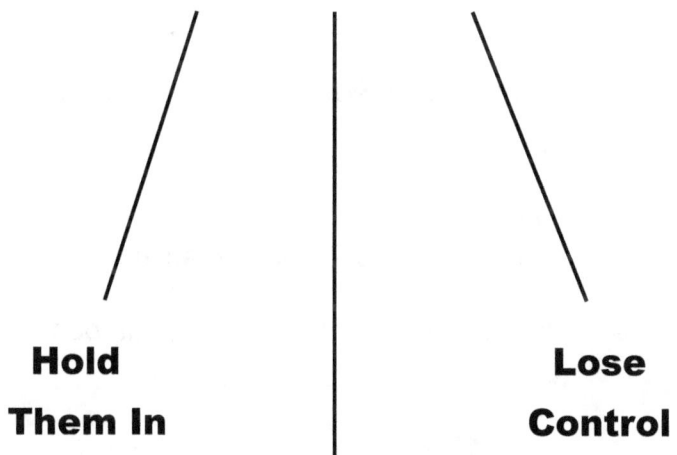

Hold Them In

Manage Them

Lose Control

So which one did you pick?

If you are a "**Manage Them**", congratulations!

You obviously know what to do with your emotions!

If you are a "**Hold Them In**",

I am going to guess at times, you also can "Lose It"!

Finally, if you start at "**Lose Control**", & stay at "Lose Control", **don't worry**! Help is on the way!

I like using a pendulum because it perfectly illustrates just how difficult can be to

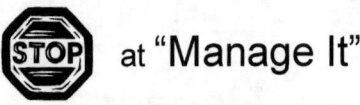 at "Manage It"

if you start up on either end.

Momentum makes it difficult to stop!

I have another way I like to teach people to think about emotions and how to manage them!

First, let me ask:

"Have you ever said something you wished had *never* come out of your mouth?"

I think most people can relate to experiences like this!!!

Here's **why it happens** –

When our emotions are so high that their level is up to our nose – simply by opening our mouth to speak they will come **SPILLING OUT!**

When things are at this high of a level – we will have **NO CONTROL** over what comes out!

Best not to say anything when emotions are this high! WAIT! There's an even worse level to be at....
BRAIN LEVEL!

When we are filled with emotion up above our 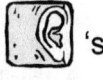 's we lose control over our brain!

It's like our brain gets **"flooded"** & we can end up
DOING STUPID THINGS,
not just saying them!

[Okay, maybe this hasn't happened to you. But I am sure you can think of other people this might describe!]

Managing emotions requires a process which has us do two things:

1) **STOP** the level from rising any higher.

2) **RELEASE SOME** so that the level will drop.

IMPORTANT:

It is only when the level is *lower* than the neck, *that we should attempt to talk!*

If our emotion is right at neck level it'll *still* **CHOKE US!**

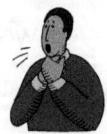

STOP the Level From Rising!

There are many ways to 🛑 our level of emotions from rising. Remember, there are both healthy AND unhealthy ways!

Think of **SURVIVAL TOOLS** vs. **LIFETOOLS!**

Some of the **unhealthy** ways: (SURVIVAL TOOLS)

Eat   Drink   Sleep   Shut down   Isolate

Avoidance   Become numb   Ignore things

Self harming behaviors   Use negative self talk

Some of the *healthy* ways: (LIFETOOLS)

Take a time out   Belly Breathing   Count to 10

Set limits   Decline to talk about it anymore

Guided Imagery   Consider the Source   Listen to music

Use the Serenity Prayer   Walk Away

Focus on something else   Use ➕ self talk

Change your thought pattern   meditation   prayer

'It is what it is'   All passive relaxation techniques

Decline the invitation to fight   walk outside & look UP!

RELEASE So the Level Will Drop

In order to **release emotion**......

muscle involvement is required.

Think of it like we are bailing water out of a boat.

We must take ACTION

in order to get the water out!

The same principle applies to emotions.

We must take ACTION to get the emotion out!

It requires we involve 'muscles'

to actually **create the release**!

The quick 3 I throw out are easy to remember:

Walk   Talk   Write!

If you remember nothing more than these & put them in to practice, you will be on your way to *managing your emotions rather than having them manage you!*

PS. You will also discover many more active releases in the next chapter on stress!
After all, emotions can often be *our response to stress!*

In my workshops, I will take a couple liter bottles 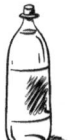 & hand them out to different people to shake them up really good.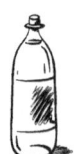

I want to use them to reinforce a point about managing emotions…….

Our **emotions** are just like the pressure that builds up inside those bottles when they get **" ALL SHOOK UP!"**

It doesn't do any good to simply ⛔ the shaking!!!!!
We must also create the release!!!

Think about it for a moment.

What happens if someone takes a bottle that's been **"ALL SHOOK UP!"** & sets it back in the refrigerator or in the cupboard?

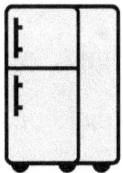 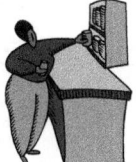

The pressure doesn't go anywhere!!!!!

UNTIL….

it just ends up dumping a mess on

the next unsuspecting person!

The same happens with our emotions….

We end up **dumping them out on the next person**!

To prevent this from happening we

MUST USE A RELEASE!

(Kind of like when you take a bottle and twist the cap a little bit at a time to let some of the pressure out!)

There is another **IMPORTANT** point to remember….

We can't often tell just by looking at the bottle whether or not it has any pressure built up inside!

Just as we often can't tell looking at a person whether or
not they have any emotional pressure built up inside!!!

The best strategy is PREVENTION! Approach with caution & be prepared to move quickly out of the way!

Stress Management Made Simple

"Raise your hand if you know STRESS is not good for your health?"

When I ask this question in my workshops – everyone in there will raise their hand! I'm sure you too would also raise your hand! So we can stop here, right? *WRONG!*

Even though we all *know* **STRESS** is *not good for us*, very few people do anything about it!

So I like to take a different approach…..

I focus on helping people 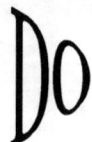 something about it!

After all,
if we can reduce our **STRESS** levels,
we can actually cut our risk of dying from
heart disease, cancer, & diabetes

I want you to get a piece of paper & pen right now, before you go to the next page.

Don't go there until you have them ready!

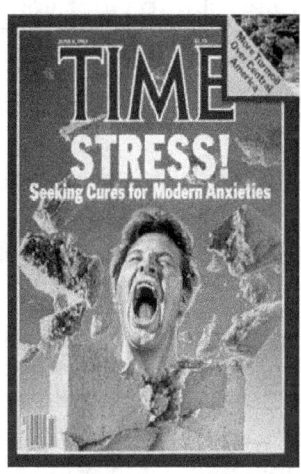

What do you think of when you see this?

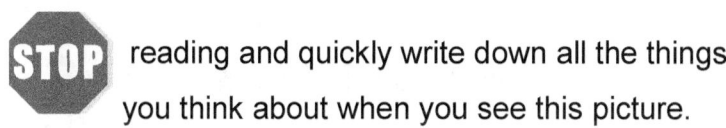 reading and quickly write down all the things you think about when you see this picture.

When you are done writing, let's continue!

I love doing this exercise! What I find is that each person usually has something different come to mind when they see or hear the word **STRESS**.

>When I do this exercise in a workshop,
>we get a lot of different answers.

>I'd like to share some of them with you!

They may be very similar to what you've written down.

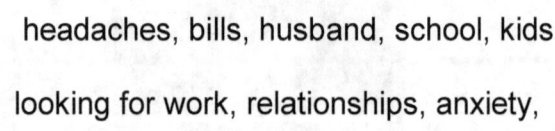

headaches, bills, husband, school, kids

looking for work, relationships, anxiety,

loss of control, can't sleep, shopping,

break up, family, job interviews, money,

birthdays, not working, overwhelmed, life, tuition,

kid's schedules, holidays, Dr.'s appointments, driving

Now here is an important part for you to understand:

What is STRESS?

"A response to a situation or change."

Let's talk about "response" for a moment.

Usually the response is something we don't

have much control over

once it starts.

Kind of like a reflex –
the doctor hits my knee and my leg moves!

Has this ever happened to you?

You have a big event going on in your life.

Let's say an interview for a job.

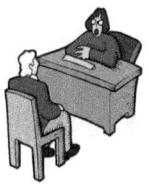

First off, you don't sleep very well the night before.

Then as you are getting ready,

your stomach starts to twist and turn.

You are about to have a case of the 'runs'!

Now, who would *actually let these responses happen*?

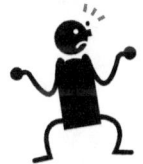

NO ONE!

This is the thing about STRESS –

Once it hits, we <u>don't</u> <u>get</u> <u>to</u> <u>have</u> too much control!

Before we move on, I also want to point out something else that is VERY important:

STRESS does not come one size fits all!

Here's what I mean by this:

1st we must realize that **'the change or situation'** does not always come in a negative form!

We can have **POSITIVE** **changes or situations** that can trigger a response.

Look at your list:

Can you identify some POSITIVE stress sources on it?

If you didn't write any down,

can you think of any right now that you could add?

2nd we must realize **'the change or situation'** does not come in just one size!

It can be either **BIG or SMALL**.

Think about it for a moment…..

What happens to your stress level when the kids are running 5 minutes late in the morning?

or

You are running 5 minutes late for an appointment?

3rd we must realize **'the change or situation'** may be stressful for one person but *not another*!

STRESS is a very **personal thing!**

Just because something may not be *STRESS to me* does not mean it *may not be STRESS to you!*

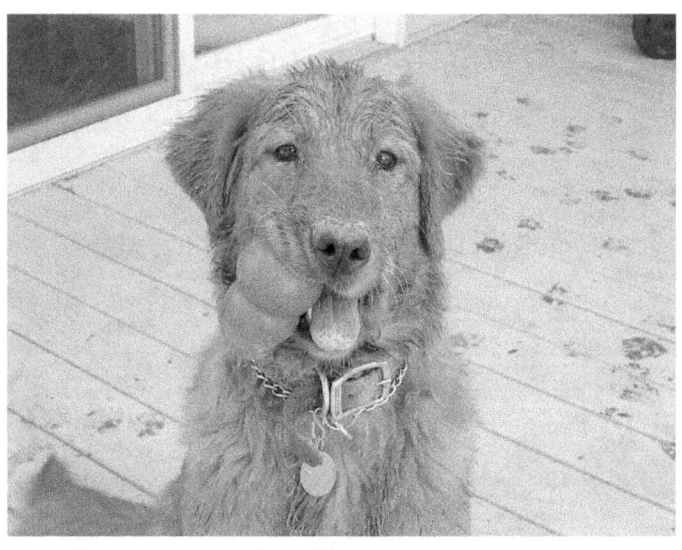

I wanted to share with you one of my
POSITIVE STRESSES!

Now that we have a little clearer picture of STRESS

LET"S DO SOMETHING ABOUT IT!!

Do you have kids?

Has your washer ever been broken?

Do you hate to do laundry?

If you answered YES to any of the above,
then you already may be a bit of a
stress expert & not even know it!

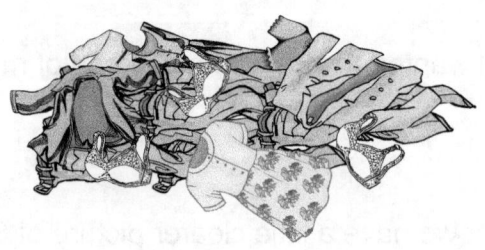

This is the pile of laundry after just 1 week!

Heading in to the next week, things are so busy that you don't have any time to do laundry. It has to **wait** until next weekend.

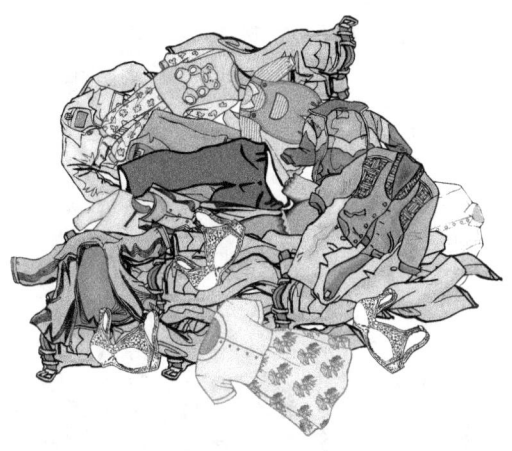

This is the pile of laundry you are looking at week 2!

It starts to GROW BIGGER!!

But wait…..

There just isn't enough time to get it all done.

You've got the kid's conference this week, it's your mother's birthday, and you still have to go shopping for a present.

Everyone has enough clothes to last them one more week…..

Besides, there isn't anything happening next weekend.

So……laundry is put off for another week!

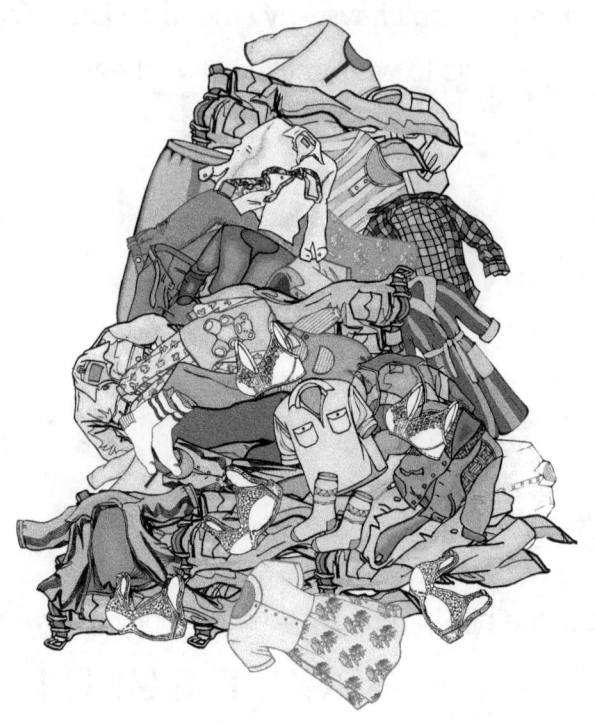

Imagine **how** you would **feel** if you had to look at a pile of laundry as tall as you?!

What can we do to *keep laundry from piling up*?

Do a load as frequently as possible!

Sometimes we may need to do **2 loads or more** a day!

STRESS is just like laundry!

It piles up!

Sure!

You can *pretend* it's not there!

Maybe even try to hide it!

Whether you see it or not –

it still keeps *piling up*!

Solution # 1:

Do **at least** one load a day of

Stress Laundry!

[This *means you must select and do at least one of the activities listed in the following pages. Don't rely on the same one or two. Try things you've never done before!*]

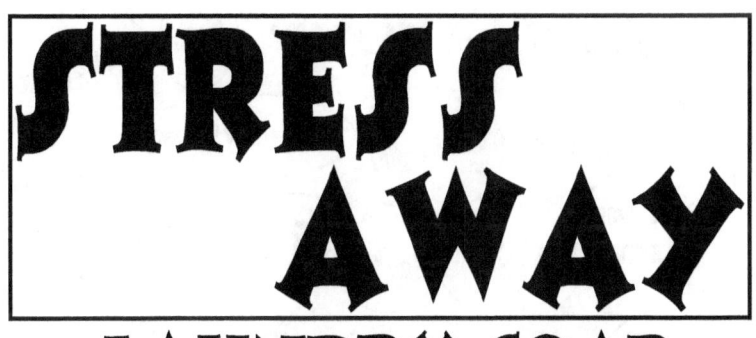

LAUNDRY SOAP

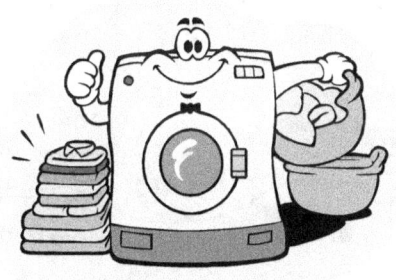

Guaranteed to lighten any day!

Directions:

* Use at least one time daily.

* Separate in to piles if too large for one load.

* May need to do multiple loads!

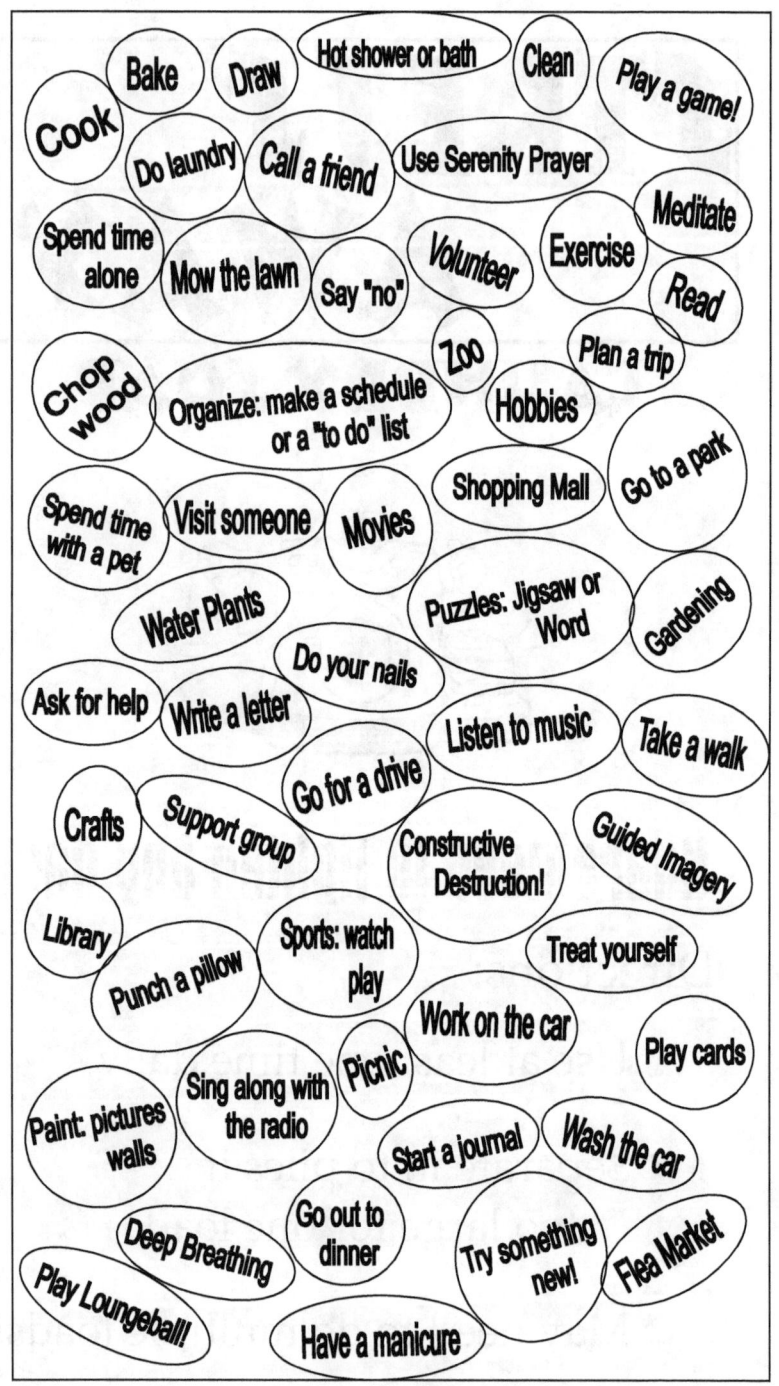

Solution # 2:

Avoid adding to the PILE!

Take steps to **AVOID** the things that cause you STRESS!

Only when I started doing my own laundry did I come to appreciate why my Mom would get so mad when I would change clothes a bunch!!

As you can see, when it comes to **STRESS**
most people are already experts!
Okay, maybe not the person who
takes everything to the dry cleaners!

It makes sense, doesn't it?

We all have to do
a little stress laundry everyday!

PS. I wanted to share some of the ways **I avoid**
adding to my pile of **STRESS**:

#1) When I have to go some place new for a speech

or an appointment, I'll go find it ahead of time.

If I can't do that,

I make sure to leave myself extra time to find it.

#2) I plan out my meals for the week & **avoid** the

STRESS of coming home from work &

trying to figure out 'what's for dinner?'

#3) At work, I **avoid** the **STRESS** of not getting things done by making sure I complete what I'm working on, before I move on to the next!

(This really use to be a **very big STRESS**, as I had this habit of skipping around to different tasks & then feeling like I wasn't accomplishing anything!)

#4) I make sure I get my exercise done each **morning** this way it's done, and I don't have to worry about still doing it when I get home from work.

However, there are many things we can't control in life.

Times in LIFE when we seem to get **DUMPED ON**.

I refer to this as

"The Dump Truck O'Stress"

Let me illustrate this next!

Dump Truck O'Stress!

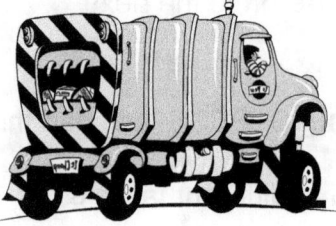

A truck full of 'dirty laundry was suddenly dropped on your front door...

How would you **FEEL**?   What would you **DO**?

Here are some pretty natural reactions:

Angry	Give Up
Overwhelmed	Explode
Powerless	Hide
Hopeless	Run

Life's big **STRESS** cause these *same reactions* –

These are life events & changes that come on quickly, without warning, and in a big way

The equivalent of a dump truck full of dirty laundry!

What to do when the Dump Truck O'Stress pulls up:

1. Give yourself permission to **feel the way you do** (Otherwise it just adds to the pile!)

2. Break it in to **smaller piles**
   (Small piles are easier to manage!)

3. Ask for **help** (The more people working on a pile, the better the chance of getting through it!)

4. Make a plan or a **time schedule**
   (This helps keep you focused!)

5. **Prioritize**
   (Figure out what's important to take care of first)

6. Be **realistic**!
   (It may take a while to chip away at the pile)

7. Take it "**one pile at a time**"
   (This makes less stress!)

The Power Tools!

WHETHER YOU THINK YOU CAN

OR

YOU THINK YOU CAN'T...

YOU'RE RIGHT!

Brain Power

One of the most powerful tools we have is our brain!

The *problem* for most people is they have theirs working **AGAINST** them instead of **FOR** them.

The previous quote says it all!
I believe it was written by Henry Ford.
(*I'm not certain as I have heard it many different times!*)

Think about it for a moment……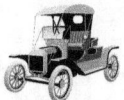

There are so many great inventors like Henry Ford, the Wright Brothers, & Thomas Edison who **thought they could**, even when *the world thought they couldn't*. In fact, the world believed it impossible!

They learned to harness their brain's power to work FOR THEM allowing their **dreams come to life!**.

I wonder?

What dreams would you achieve if **you believed YOU COULD!!!!!!**

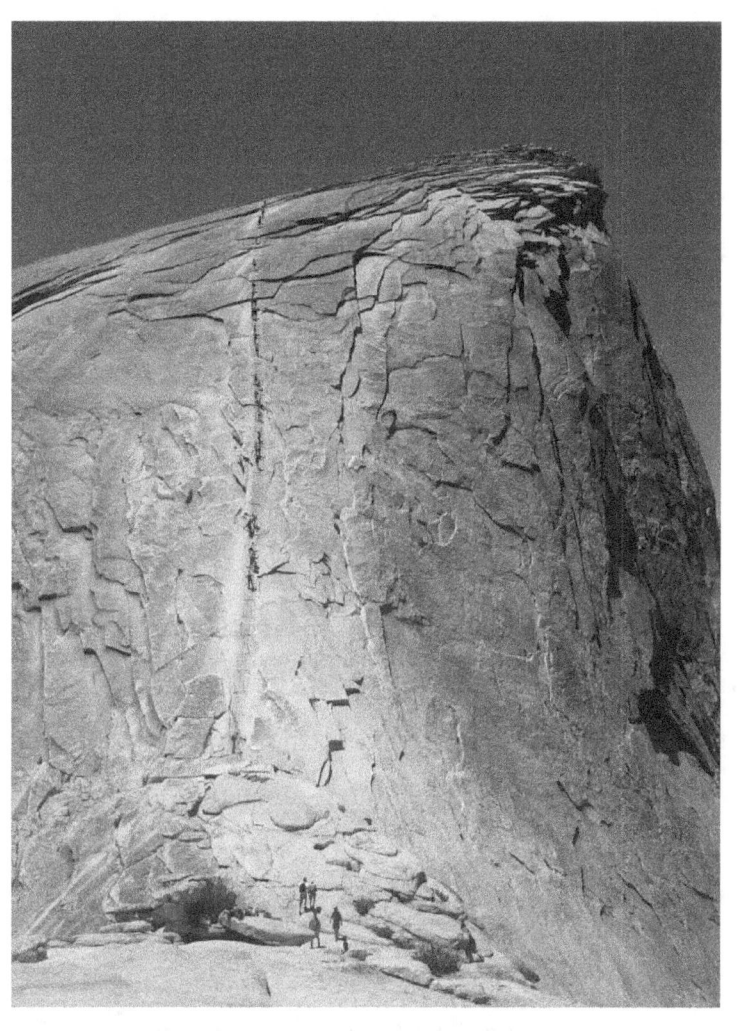

This is my example of:

"If you think you can or you think you can't, You're right"

This is Half Dome, located in *Yosemite National Park*. This is a view that **most** of the park's millions of visitors each year will **NEVER** see.....

In order to get where this picture was taken, you have to hike **8 miles** in to the *back country* of Yosemite.

Of course, it's all up hill! It ends up rising from 4,000 foot elevation in the valley to 8,800 feet at the top.

My brother & I had reached the bottom of the dome. I can't repeat exactly what he said, but a clean translation is "Holy Shit!" At that moment our thoughts of climbing to the top vanished! However, we felt very proud of our accomplishment just getting to here!

We didn't think we could!

My nieces unexpectedly showed up! We thought they were ahead of us & half way up the dome by now! Excited & eager for us to ALL reach the top, they encouraged us to give it a try. After all, we had come this far.....

They got us thinking we could!

And we did!

This is the view from the top!

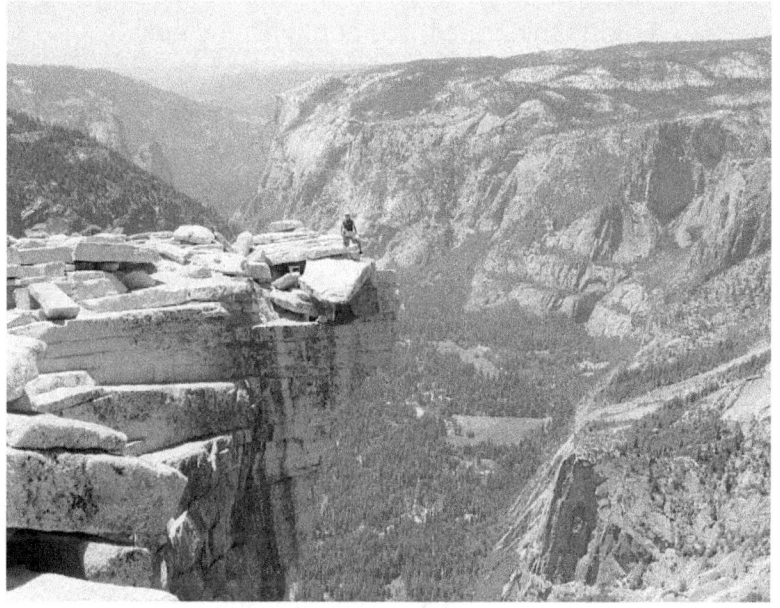

Yosemite Valley is down below!

I don't know who the guy was!
I just thought he was brave.

What are YOU stopping yourself from doing?!

A Life Changed

It comes as quite a shock to my patients & colleagues I *was once* the **most negative, pessimistic person!**

I didn't think anything could go my way.

I was working **12** hours a day and

still barely paying my bills.

I made **less** at my job than what I paid to go to college. For me, there was *nothing good about anything.*

But then in 1989 I had a moment that was life changing. I will share more about this in a moment. Since then, I've tried to learn as much as I can about using the power of thoughts as a tool for transformation & wellness. My study has impacted both my personal and professional life. As I learn new ideas & strategies, I try to incorporate them not only in to my life but also in to my work with others. After all, what good is knowledge if it is not shared! I'm on a mission to share what I have learned with others!

I'm thankful for the opportunity to share it with you.

I had mentioned earlier that I had a moment in 1989
which changed my life around.

It was a blessing hidden in heart ache.

&
has truly shaped the life I live today.

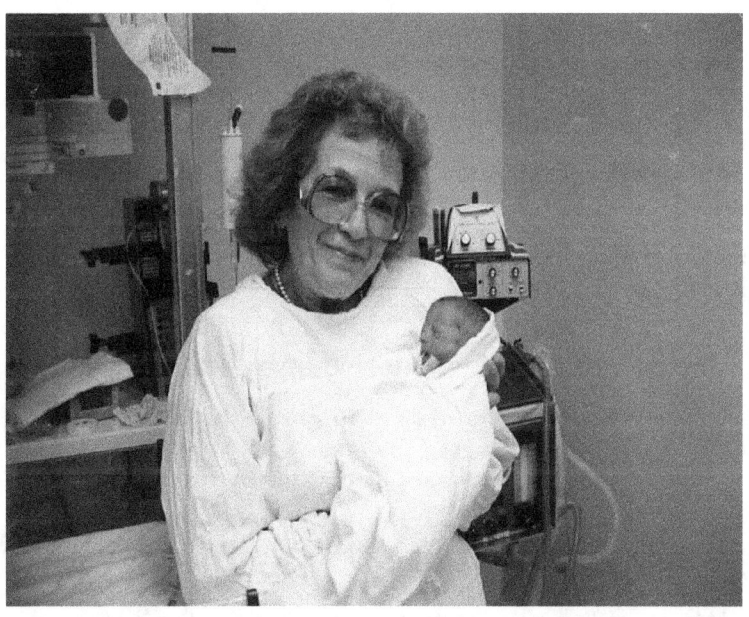

This is a picture of my mother taken December, 1988.
She is holding my nephew, Christopher.

It is my mother who gave me
the greatest gift a person could receive.
Let me explain…..

My mother had called me at work to tell me her doctor wanted her to come in to the hospital right away. It was only when we got in to a room at the emergency room my mother finally told me about the **cancer**.

It is *no surprise* she had kept this information to herself. After all, she'd done it before.

That afternoon I was on the phone with my sisters out in California making plans to get my mother out West so she could have a chance to see everyone.

Those plans <u>never</u> <u>happened</u>……..

My mother ended up passing away that very night. With the tears, sadness, grief and heartache came the greatest gift I could ever receive:

It doesn't matter what we plan for tomorrow ~
We must live our life today as if it were the only one.

We must live One Day At A Time

I like to share the **power of serenity** that goes along with being able to live one day at a time.

I have an exercise I created & I'd like to share with you.

First, read the following:

YESTERDAY, TODAY, and TOMORROW

There are two days in every week that we need not worry about, two days that must be kept free from fear and apprehension.

One is **YESTERDAY**, with it's mistakes & cares, it's faults & blunders, it's aches & pains. Yesterday has passed, forever beyond our control. All the money in the world cannot bring back yesterday. We cannot undo a single act we performed. Nor can we erase a single word we've said – Yesterday is gone!

The other day we must not worry about is **TOMORROW**, with it's impossible adversaries, it's burden, it's hopeful promise and poor performance. Tomorrow is beyond our control!

Tomorrow's sun will rise either in splendor or behind a mask of clouds – but it will rise. And until it does, we have no stake in tomorrow, for it is yet unborn.

This leaves only one day – **TODAY**. Any person can fight the battles of just one day. It is only when we add the burdens of yesterday & tomorrow that we break down.

It is not the experience of today that drives people mad—it is the remorse of bitterness for something which happened yesterday, and the dread of what tomorrow may bring. <u>LET US LIVE ONE DAY AT A TIME!!!!</u>

(Author Unknown)

Second, take a blank piece of paper and
write Yesterday, Tomorrow, & Today on it
so it looks like this:

```
┌─────────────────────────┐
│        Yesterday        │
│                         │
│                         │
│        Tomorrow         │
│                         │
│                         │
│         Today           │
│                         │
│                         │
└─────────────────────────┘
```

Under "Yesterday" -

I want you to write down all the things from **the past** (from yesterday or 20 years ago) that still occupy your thoughts. This includes regrets, resentments, hurts, the I shoulda-woulda-coulda's, guilt's, & anything else!

Under Tomorrow -

I want you to write down all the things from **the future** that occupy your thoughts. This includes worries, fears, "what-if's", uncertainties, hopes, & dreams!

Under TODAY -

I want you to look back over the things you've written under yesterday & tomorrow. Ask yourself this **?** about *each* of the items you have listed:

"Is there anything I can DO about that TODAY?"

If there is, write down under **TODAY** the **SPECIFIC ACTION** you can take.

It must be something you can DO!

If there isn't,
don't write anything under TODAY

Once you have completed this,
there is one last step to take!

Fold the paper *just above* where **TODAY** is written.

Now, keep folding it back & forth several times on that same crease. You can even lick it if you want but don't get a paper cut!

Now carefully **tear the paper along the crease**.

DO NOT USE SCiSSORS!!!

It is IMPORTANT to do it by your own hand.

You should end up with 2 pieces of paper in your hands.

One piece has Yesterday & Tomorrow on it.

Feel free to burn this, rip it up, shred it, and destroy it!

The other piece has TODAY on it.

Hold onto this!

It is the only day we CAN do anything about.

You may need to do repeat this every day until you're able to focus on TODAY!

Another way of looking at it:

'WHY's'

GET US LOST IN THE PAST

'WHAT-IF's'

GET US LOST IN THE FUTURE

CAROL L RICKARD

Are these words you often speak?

If so, they will prevent you from

Living in Today!

One More Power Tool

Another *powerful* **LIFETOOL** for me has long been the Serenity Prayer. I started putting it in to practice in my life after I started working an addictions treatment unit.

I had heard of & was familiar with it; however it wasn't until I was around people who could teach me how to USE IT, that it became one of my primary tools. Just like 'One Day at a Time' - this **LIFETOOL** holds

The Power of Peace & Serenity

My strongest test of this tool came in the summer of 2006. It was in July when my sister Kris suddenly died.

Since I live in central New Jersey, I flew out of Philadelphia. My flight got out of the gate right on time....but once on the way to the runway; we sat there for almost **2** hours.

I was to catch a connecting flight out of Salt Lake City in to Reno. My brother & his family, flying from

Virginia, were on the same flight out of Salt Lake City. Needless to say – I never caught up with them.

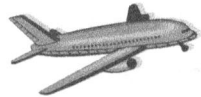

My delay in Philly had me miss the connecting flight. The worst news came when I was booked on a flight the next morning: **1 hour** after the funeral was to start. Now here I was stranded the night in Salt Lake City.

Really, what could I do? So, I kept the Serenity Prayer repeating in my head over & over & over again.

I called my family from the airport in Salt Lake City & informed them I wouldn't even be leaving Salt Lake City
**until the next day and
AFTER the funeral had already started.**

As I kept repeating the Serenity Prayer, I let the tears flow. I had a lot of mixed emotions and I knew it wasn't a good idea to hold them in.

In the past, under stressful conditions like these I would have had a major migraine before the plane ever landed in Utah.

Turns out, I didn't get a migraine all weekend. This was despite not getting to my sister's house until AFTER all the days events had taken place. My **LIFETOOL** held me steady!

As I said a little earlier in this book, there are many times in life we don't get to choose what happens.....

We *DO* get to *CHOOSE* our *RESPONSE* to them!

God grant me,

The *Serenity* to accept the things I cannot change

The *Courage* to change the things I can

And the *Wisdom* to know the difference

Here is my shortened version of it:

Can I do anything about it right now?

If not, I just have to **let it go!**

Important:

I would like to make this point about *'Letting Go'* or as they say in recovery circles: *'Let go and let God'*

We cannot let go of something we have not allowed ourselves to feel!

In order to 'let go' of something –

we must first **FEEL the FEELINGS** connected to it

and then

'Let Go'!

(One way to think of this is we simply have something come in through one ear, acknowledge it (feel it!), and move on out through the other side!)

Another way I explain 'Let Go' to my patients:

Leave

Everything

To

Gods

Ownership

© 2016 & licensed by Well YOUniversity, LLC
Taken from "Words At Work"

And one last way to practice "Letting Go"!

Write down what it is you are trying to 'let go' of on a small slip of paper.

Then do one of the following with the slip:

✶ **Put it in a special box you have decorated**
(Many people refer to these as a God Box or a Worry Box. You can find all types of boxes at your local craft store)

✶ **Put it in a special book**
(This could be a book of worship or another special book of yours)

✶ **Throw it in a fireplace**
(If you don't have one, it could be any other safe way to destroy it by burning!)

✶ **Shred it up**
(This could be as simple as throwing it in the shredder or tearing it by hand in to a bunch of little itty, bitty pieces!

You will notice the one thing these all have in common
is they **REQUIRE ACTION BE TAKEN!**
Instead of just trying to do this '*all in our head*',
we get our entire body involved in the process!

I believe it is this **PRINCIPLE OF DOING**
which leads us to great success.

When our mind starts to go back
to thinking about it again…..

Be prepared that it will!
Our mind <u>will</u> try to hold on to things!!

We can also remind ourselves we have "gotten rid"
of **what** it is trying to access again!

Wrapping Things Up

We started off by taking a look at how we can
USE FOOD AS A SURVIVAL TOOL. My hope is you
now have a better understanding of the behavior &
instead of beating yourself up over it; you can
validate the important role it ONCE played in your life.

2 questions to now ask yourself:

Is this **SURVIVAL TOOL** now hurting me?
Is it time for me to turn in my **SURVIVAL TOOLS?**

If the answer is **NO**, that's okay!
Now just may not be the time for you to do so.

We all have our own journey to take us
to a point where it is time to change.

As long as you are honest with yourself
& promise to re-visit this question,
I hold on to the hope that when the
time comes for you to change,

YOU WILL!

If the answer is **YES**,

I hold on to the hope that you may now have enough **"LIFETOOLS'** to get the job done!

Remember, learning anything new requires practice for it to become a new habit. Change is a process!!

Do not get discouraged should you find yourself slipping back to old behaviors every now & then. Learn from the 'slips' and move on.

Two steps forward, one step back still has us moving closer to our goals.

Try this exercise!

Start on one side of a room.
Take two steps forward & one step back.
Now, do it again!
Two steps forward & one step back.

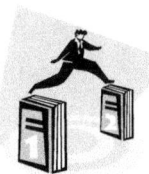

Repeat this process at least 2 more times!

Are you closer to the other side
of the room than where you started?

YES!!!

So when your brain starts to yell at you:
'you're going backwards' Yell back! "No I'm not!!"

The next area we focused on:
CAROL'S LAWS OF LASTING WAIST LOSS

Okay, it was Weight Loss, but
you know how I feel about this word!!

Keep thinking of your body as a car!

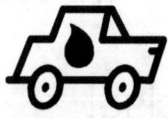

Don't overfill the **GAS TANK**!

Keep the **ENGINE** running!

Be sure to use the right **KINDS OF GAS**!

Pull from the **SPARE TANKS**!

These laws will not fail you!

The third area we focused on:
IS IT REALLY HUNGER

The goal here is you start becoming aware of

WHY

you are putting that food in your mouth!

Is it physical hunger or emotional hunger?

Step 1 - use the guidelines we talked about to help you figure this out.

Step 2 - do one of the following:

Feed physical hunger something healthy!
or
Feel the emotions & then release them.

Again, since this is new,
it may take some practice for you to get better at it!!

Don't beat yourself up if you stumble.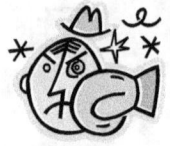

We then focused on:
STRESS. MANAGEMENT MADE SIMPLE!

The goal here is to have gotten you thinking differently about STRESS & seeing how easy it is to do something about it!

Remember, the best way to stress less is
DO A LOAD OF STRESS LAUNDRY EVERDAY!

As you become more aware of when it is
PILING UP,

You may need to do extra loads!

And of course, the BEST strategy is to
avoid adding to the pile in the first place.

Be on the look out:
STRESS comes in all shapes & sizes!

The last area we focused on: **THE POWER TOOLS**.

Once you can get your brain working
for you rather than against you –

YOU CAN ACCOMPLISH ANYTHING!

Our thoughts & the words we choose to use
are the paint brushes we use to create our life!

If you take nothing else away from this chapter
I can only hope that it is how to use

One Day at A Time
&
The Serenity Prayer

CHECK OUT THE SPECIAL BONUS ON THE NEXT PAGE!

A BONUS GIFT!

We have a special bonus for you!

Go to:

www.StopUsingFoodToCope.com/blueprint

Put your name and email in the box
Click "Send Me My Blueprint Carol!"

Once you have confirmed it is okay to add you to our email server, we will send you an email containing **our secret blueprint for success**!

Be on the lookout -
It will come from Well YOUniversity!

You can always reach us at:
Success@WellYOUniversity.com

www.ingramcontent.com/pod-product-compliance
Lightning Source LLC
LaVergne TN
LVHW051845080426
835512LV00018B/3076